The Chiology way to happiness.

Uzoma Chika N. Nwosu, MD

(An Igbo approach to happiness.)

Manufactured in the United States.

Library of Congress catalogue in-
publication data. Nwosu, Uzoma Chika

Edited by Kelechi Njoku

The Chiology way to happiness.

Author: Uzoma Nwosu, M.D.

Key Words: 1.Chi 2. Chiology 3. Way 4.
Happiness.5. Coherent breathing 6. Movement
7. Heavens 8. Healthy Lifestyle

This book is not intended to be used as a substitute for medical advice and treatment.

Always look up words you do not understand in a Standard English dictionary.

Table of Contents

Acknowledgements.

Many thanks to the ancient Igbos and all people who speak Igbo.

Preface

This book is a common sense approach to the pursuit of happiness based on ancient and current Igbo culture. It primarily focuses on the Chi-the personal guardian of an individual. By using breathing and movement techniques, an individual could increase their level of happiness, while eliminating negative emotions such as sadness and anger.

This book is intended to be a bridge to a higher level and quality of living.

I strongly believe that this book could help:

- Breath work practitioners.
- Anthropologists
- Igbo scholars
- Igbo linguists
- Christians
- Practitioners of other religions.
- Healers.
- Teachers
- And a host of other professionals.

This book is not intended to promote fortune telling. Fear is one of the reasons preventing knowledgeable individuals from writing a book like this. This book is intended to help you overcome fear so you can have more love and happiness.

Most of the information in this book is well known but it can be considered a new creation. The word 'ke' which means to create is also the same word for to 'bind' or 'string together'. This book is an artistic 'binding together' of mostly known facts.

The purpose of Chiology is to help spread love and happiness around the world. This can help bring people together, encourage world peace, and allow us to eliminate weapons of mass destruction.

Happiness

Happiness can be considered as a state of physical and mental well-being. A happy person can be considered to be in good social standing with many of their goals achieved, and with many achievable future goals. A happy person can be associated with the emotion happiness and love. The pursuit of happiness is a frequent topic that humans are interested in and actively seek.

In a rapidly changing world, happiness has become a challenge for many. Many struggle to achieve their target goals and objectives, and this can lead to frustration and unhappiness.

In Igbo when someone is happy they could say "obi di mụ mma". Literally, 'obi di mụ mma' means 'heart is good to my soul'. A person who is happy has a good heart that is good to an individual's soul. Not surprisingly, happiness has been linked to longevity. A happy person is likely to be good to other souls as well. It would seem like one of the benefits of the state of happiness is soul nourishment. On the other hand, an unhappy person stresses their soul. This is one of the reasons people strive to be happy, and why happiness is a good thing.

In Igbo, 'arụ mụ' refers to 'my body', while 'mụ' is my soul. 'Mụ' is also the word for 'learn'. As if it was not enough, 'mụ' is also the word for 'smile'. The link between a smile and happiness does not need further emphasis.

So 'mụ'=my soul= learn=smile. This is because the soul is used in learning. The soul is used in assessing and making life decisions that can bring more success and happiness.

When an individual is happy, their soul functions better and provides more accurate answers. The opposite happens in unhappiness, sadness, depression and similar conditions.

Happiness is not possible when we are not learning. Some philosophers believe that happiness is a condition in which an individual has learned the knowhow to overcome future obstacles.

Happiness has been described as covering a spectrum of emotions ranging from contentment to joy. Enjoyment can be viewed as a higher form of happiness. Coining the word for enjoyment must have been challenging for the ancient people, but they settled on 'añụli'. 'Añụli' was coined from 'añụ' which refers to 'honey' and 'li' which we can loosely translate to as 'imbibe or eat'.

Hopefully, these Chiology steps would bring you close to the emotion associated with 'eating honey'.

Chiology

Chiology was coined from 'Chi' (personal guide) and 'logy' (study). Chiology is the study of the Chi. All Chiologists are students of the 'Chi'. This work focuses on the Chi which was called by the author Chinua Achebe as the "personal god of an individual". It is believed that it is not possible to completely know the Chi hence the phrase 'amama amasi amasi' and 'Chiebuka' (The Chi is very big). The Chi is closely related to the concept of God which is known as Chukwu (Chi-ukwu or Big Chi).

Chiology is non-religious but can be considered a cultural approach to happiness. Mentions of God, and the concept of God, in this work should not be misinterpreted as suggesting that Chiology is a religion. Life in ancient Igbo was constructed from a God concept and it is impossible to entirely separate man from the God concept in Igbo. Whenever possible, the concept of God will be referred to as the Big Chi.

The Chiological way to happiness is based on the Igbo concept of the Chi. The Chi is a force that determines the destiny of an individual. Some authors have called the Chi an individuals personal god, others have referred to the Chi as a personal spiritual guardian. The Chi predicts success and failures. When an individual experiences a misfortune, the Chi is responsible.

In Igbo every individual has a spirit called 'mmụọ'. They also have a soul called 'mụ' and a body called 'arụ mụ'. Apparently, the soul is encapsulated by the body. In Chiology, it is understood that your spirit (not your body) is reading this book. The soul is helping the spirit relate the words to other knowledge in the current world.

In addition, every individual has a Chi. The Chi is intimately related to the soul 'mụ'.

An individual's Chi, leads the individual, hence the statement 'Chibụzọ'. When an individual wakes up in the morning, his/her Chi is already there waiting.

The Igbo

Igbo is the name given to an ethnic group whose primary homeland is in South Eastern Nigeria. Based on archeological evidence, Igbos have lived in their current homeland for thousands of years. They speak the Igbo language which is verb based. Igbo was coined from the verb 'gbo' which means to 'prevent' or 'guard'. That same verb is seen in the word for farming 'ugbo' and in the word 'egbo' which is a group of specialized trees used as a fence. Farming and fencing are preventive measures against hunger and intruders respectively. The 'i', 'e' and 'u' in 'Igbo', 'egbo' and 'ugbo' are prefixes used to modify the meaning of a verb. For details on Igbo prefixes and suffixes, please find the book 'Igbo voices; hidden wisdom from an ancient language" or "Chi, and healing words from an ancient language".

One of the ways of being an Igbo person is to assume the stance of a guard. Igbos are known to go to incredible lengths to have money in an effort to guard against poverty.

Ancient Igbos did a terrific job creating their language in order to maximize communication accuracy.

> **Important Notice**: The Igbo language is verb based. Actions were translated into verbs that are identified by their sound. There are some verbs that sound phonologically slightly different from each other. These verbs represent similar actions. The difference could be because the activities are performed in different environments, e.g. in the physical or spiritual planes. It can also be due to the presence of prefixes or suffixes that modify the sound of the verb. For example, the word Iwe (anger) is derived from

'we' which means to 'withdraw'. The 'we' in 'Iwe' is slightly different phonologically. However, both sounds convey similar actions because anger is a 'withdrawal'. This is why it is difficult to talk to an angry person.

The Igbo methodical approach in preventing unhappiness and misfortune is legendary.

This book is intended to introduce you to some of the ancient methods.

The Chi

To understand the Chi better, I would like to show you circumstances in which Chi is used in the Igbo language.

Igbo is a verb based language. Words are constructed from verbs which are action words. In the physical universe, humans have goals and purposes which require action. The ancient Igbos translated actions into words. Similar actions are represented by similar words. For example, the word for 'leg' (ụkwụ) shares the same verb 'kwụ' with the word for 'stand' (kwụ)-the leg is used for standing.

Verbs were used to construct words for a very practical reason-competence in actions is the basis of happiness. By understanding and knowing words, an individual can gain competence in the actual actions.

These are some words that have Chi in them:

Igbo	English	Comments
Chukwu (Chi-ukwu)	God	God is the Big Chi.
Chineke	God	Chi creates. Chi is the creator. To create something you have to bring different things together.
Chi	Chi	Personal guardian of an individual. Determines the destiny of an individual.
Chi mụ	My Chi	Chi mụ can be more accurately described as the 'Chi of my soul'.

		'mu' is my soul, while 'aru mu' is my body or body of my soul.
Mme-chi	Closing	More accurately, it means to approximate, or bring together. To close a door is to bring its edges together.
Chi, Chi-e	Rub	In the action of rubbing, one is bringing two things together. One is bringing items into a 'head'.
Uzoechina	Let the road not close.	They actual mean, let the road not approximate-or let the road not end.
Nti ichi	Deafness	Deafness was considered closing or approximation of the ears.
Chi-Jii	Nightfall, darkness	Night is an ending or approximation. Like the 'fall of the curtain' for the show the sun put up during the day. Chi-jii can be translated as the 'Chi has darkened'.
Chi fo	New day	Day is an unfolding of the end. The cycles of day and night are related to an individual's Chi. After all, actions and counter actions

17

		happen either during the day or at night. Generally speaking, more activities are performed during the day.

We can readily notice that an individual has a Chi, and God is the Big Chi. God is love and love can be considered as a force that brings entities together. An individual's Chi could be considered their 'end', where their being 'approximates', or where they come to a 'head'. This is their control center or their 'cockpit'.

'Chi mụ' is a short phrase that is understood as 'my Chi'. However, it should be understood as the 'Chi of my soul'. Since Chi means to bring together, to 'end', or approximate; 'Chi mụ' should be understood as "the end of my soul" or "where my soul comes together". If the soul were an apple, then its Chi is where the apple connects to a supplying branch.

The Chi is a very complex subject but we can loosely state that the Chi is a force that brings an individual together with his environment. It is a force that acts to bring an individual together with himself/herself, his God, other people, animals and plants, and other entities in the physical universe. Chinua Achebe describes it as the "personal god of an individual" while others have called it the 'life force of an individual'.

We know from Psychology and related disciplines that negative emotions such as stress, sadness, anger, grief, jealousy, revenge etc, leads to destructive thoughts and actions. On the other hand, positive emotions such as love and happiness lead to more positive actions. Since God (Big Chi) is love, Chiology can be considered as a series of steps to bring an individual to the state of love. Chiology is about bringing an individual close to his/her Chi and the 'Big Chi'. The anticipated result is more love and happiness. Chiology can be considered the war of love and happiness.

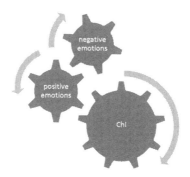

The Chi: negative emotions such as anger and frustration work against the Chi.

Some of the properties of the Chi are:

Characteristic	Comments
Chi-di-ebele	The Chi is merciful. One of the properties of the Chi is mercy. A person with a good Chi shows mercy to the poor, handicapped, weak and the underprivileged.
Onye kwe chi ya ekwe	When one agrees, his/her Chi also agrees. When one creates agreements or bonds, the Chi would come along.
Chi mụ anya	The Chi is awake. One of the properties of the Chi is alertness or wakefulness.
Chi-fụ	The Chi sees. The Chi could see what our eyes cannot see.
Chi-ma	The Chi knows. The Chi contains knowledge that can be used by an

	individual to solve daily problems.
Chi-ji-ndụ	Chi is the holder of the energy of life. A person who is not aware and does not nourish their Chi may not be fully alive. Such as person may just be a body (arụ).
Chi-wetalụ/Chi-nyelụ	Ultimately the Chi brings all the things we have. People that are wealthy could have 'bigger' Chi. When we receive good things from people, we should consider the possibility that it's their Chi that gave us.
Chi mụ egbuo mụ	My Chi has killed me. This may be hard to swallow, but anytime an individual faces a misfortune, the Chi is to blame.
Ife si na Chi	Things come from the Chi. This suggests that good and bad things come from the Chi. Whatever the condition of an individual, it is their Chi. The Chi makes a person a musician, a teacher or a billionaire.
Chi-gbo	The Chi can prevent misfortune.
Chi-nụa Chi- nụalụmọgụ	The Chi fights or the Chi can fight for me. Some authors have described life as a struggle, suggesting that we need to fight to get what we want. However, while we are busy relaxing and sipping tea, we can score something big or record great success. The Chi is responsible for bringing us good fortune. It also means that the Chi can fight for me and thwart the plans of the enemy.
Chi-ka	The Chi is greater. The Chi is greater than anything you can imagine including diamonds and luxury cars.

The Chiology way.

These are a series of steps that could bring more happiness and love. They are based on concepts of Igbo language and culture.

These concepts are often captured as names. Ideally, an individual takes a stand in the community based on their name. They should be a resource regarding the concept the 'name' describes. In other words, they should have more than general knowledge of the principles and practices associated with their names. Name is known as 'afa'. Afa is derived from 'fa' which is 'them' or 'others'. The sound 'a' is used to reverse the notion of 'them'-a name is unique and separates an individual from other members of the community.

This section talks about Chiology way. This can also be called the Chiology steps. We can readily note that 'steps' and 'way' can be used interchangeably. In Igbo, the word for a 'way' is called 'Uzọ'. 'Uzọ' is derived from the verb 'zọ' which is to 'step'. This is because a 'way' comes about by 'steps'. This is obvious when you visit a village anywhere in the world where the villagers create 'paths' through their 'steps'. The lesson here is that each time we are stepping, we are creating a way.

Now 'zọ' also means to 'save'. This is because each time we take a 'step', we 'save' our feet on the ground. Physically speaking, what creates a way is our 'saved steps'. This is what kills the grass or moves the ground. This can be obvious when we walk on a sandy beach and notice we have saved our feet behind. Further, each step works to save us from falling. Just imagine a baby learning to walk and how important each step is.

So we can readily understand that a way is 'steps' and is also 'saving'. In reality, a "way" saves us time and minimizes danger.

21

The I-95 from New York to Boston is intended to save time and lives.

The Chiological way are steps that can save you time and could prevent misfortune. They are intended to save you from sorrow and mishap so you can have more love and happiness.

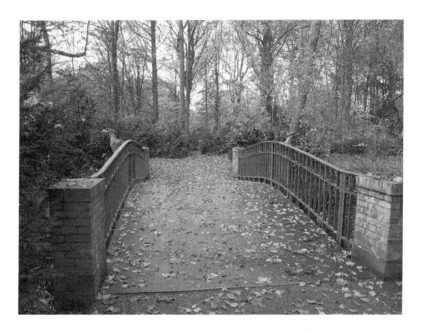

The way to happiness and freedom. Image by Lienhard Schulz.

The Way

Step 1   Chibuzo (Chi is first)

The first step in Chiology is putting the Chi first. The concept of God is understood as the 'Big Chi'. The Big Chi is the Big Love. In ideal circumstances, an individual's Chi should contain pure love and that can make a person like a god (an entity with immense creative powers).

One of the most strategic re-arrangement an individual can make is putting the Chi first. The purpose is to align an individual to love. Love is a beautiful emotion that gives an individual clarity of thought which could lead to more power over their environment. Love is more powerful than negative emotions such as fear and doubt.

In this step, an individual does whatever is necessary to align their Chi to love. When an individual wakes up, their Chi is their waiting. Some people read the bible, sing praises or pray as a way to reconnect to love or the 'Big Chi'. Others participate in meditation exercises or practice breathing meditation. Some take to physical activity like dancing, jogging, running or lifting weights.

The purpose is to remove negative emotions from the Chi, so love can prevail. This is a good way to start the day.

'Chibụzọ' means 'Chi is the first' but it also means 'Chi is the way'.

This is because, 'ibụzọ', which refers to 'being first' is also 'being the way'. The 'first' man to step on the moon has opened a 'way' for other men to step on the moon.

23

In the real world, people face temptations that can be quite risky. 'Chibuzo' demands that the Chi should be considered before one takes any risky actions.

Dangerous actions that can lead to injury and bring down the emotional level should be avoided.

Summary

The first step in Chiology is to put the Chi first. Activities such as Bible study, prayer, praise singing, dancing, jogging, etc are recommended to connect the Chi to love.

Another important step in Chiology is to realize the Chi as the guide. It may not be possible to physically locate the Chi in the human body but rest assured that it exists. There is the phrase 'Chidi' which suggests that the 'Chi exists'. There is no doubt that the Chi exists. If you are wearing a red shirt, just note that your Chi made you wear a red shirt. Even an individual in prison wearing what they do not want- it is still the Chi that is responsible. In the latter case, the Chi has brought misfortune.

An understanding of the Chi as the guide is intended to reinforce the awareness of one's Chi. This can be done by awareness of an individual's emotions. This is very common sense.

When an individual wakes up sad, and is always unhappy at work, it is time to get help. Someone with unhappiness or sadness in their Chi would most probably go downhill. If nothing is done, they are likely to have a bleak future at work and in their relationships.

An individual who is aware of the Chi, who meets someone that elicits a negative emotion, knows that something is wrong. Individuals are known to flash anger or fear at the sight of certain individuals even in the absence of provocation. Sometimes these are individuals they know, other times they are new individuals. In such cases, their Chi could be signaling some information to them. Sometimes, the Chi is requesting that we confront a certain person, but knowledge or expertise is required to address a situation appropriately.

There have been cases of individuals who planned to enter a certain vehicle but receive information from their Chi not to get in. These individuals would later learn that the vehicle was involved in a deadly accident. These are cases of Chi-nazọ (the Chi saves) or Chi-gbo (the Chi guards).

For an individual, there are places or items that can bring down their emotions. An old car, because of a fear of a break down, can cause emotional disturbances in an individual. The common sense solution in this case is, off-course, to work towards replacing the car.

For some people, food or medicines can be a culprit. There are foods that can cause intestinal upset. In this case, the gut sends messages to the brain that something is wrong. Sometimes the offending agent can be milk, especially in patients with lactase deficiency. (Lactase is an enzyme that breaks down lactose in milk). The common sense solution to this is to remove or reduce the amount of milk in the diet. Additional measures can also be taken.

Summary

Let your Chi be your guide. Be more aware of your emotions, and let them be your guide. Avoid or handle situations that weaken the Chi.

If you know plenty of Igbos, chances are you'd come across someone named 'Mmadụabụchi'. 'Mmadụabụchi' is often shortened into 'Abụchi' and represents the phrase 'man is not the Chi'.

Every human being has a Chi, the life force of an individual that determines their actions and destiny.

In the real world, people are often oppressed in their countries, in work places, in relationships and in many other circumstances. In such circumstances, an individual's Chi can be usurped by another person. It could be a manager or a superior at work.

This explains why unhappiness is very rife in work places. An individual cannot be happy and loving when their Chi has been taken over by another person.

As a student or an employee, one may have to go through emotionally challenging situations to make it to the next level. This can be considered a necessary sacrifice. However, when one gets out of school or work, at the end of the day, it might be necessary to regain their connectedness to their Chi.

Mmadụabụchi (man is not the Chi) is a statement of defiance. In Chiology, it is one of the most important ways of being. Defiance to the idea that another human being can takeover and control another individuals Chi indefinitely.

In the world, different groups of people are oppressed. In the United States, African Americans were heavily oppressed until the Civil Rights Movement brought some relief. The Igbo people were brutalized during the Nigerian civil war and for many years thereafter. Among the Igbos, there are the Osus or outcasts who are humiliated, treated like lepers, exploited, marginalized and robbed in daylight with impunity.

The concept of 'Iloabuchi' (the postulate that..*(man)..* is not the Chi) was introduced to help people embed 'man is not the Chi' into their 'spirit' and Chi. This could be done by repeating the following phrases multiple times: "man is not the Chi, a person is not the Chi,...not the Chi". (repeat as often as necessary). A Christian could consider stating that-"Jesus is my Chi". Iloabuchi is a way to defy oppression.

The word to oppress someone was coined as 'mmegbu'. 'Mme' is the word 'to make' while 'gbu' is 'to kill'. Many oppressors are not aware that their actions kill the spirit, soul, body and the Chi of the oppressed. Although there are groups such as masochists who reportedly obtain pleasure from pain, but this can be considered unusual. Again, Iloabuchi is used to help an individual confront and handle oppressive situations.

There are two possible ways to handle an oppressor. One way is to confront the oppressor. Off-course, an individual needs some tact to achieve this. It may be safer to confront an oppressor on smaller issues before tackling bigger ones. However, one must recognize that there are oppressors that cannot be easily confronted. For example, a concentration camp inmate cannot easily confront Adolf Hitler or his SS Guards. The other way to handle an oppressor is to flee or escape. In Igbo, it is termed 'ọsọndu' or "running for your life". This is not cowardly in any way. When a crazed individual has usurped and is maiming another's Chi, it is reasonable to 'escape' the oppressor. Many Jews who escaped the Nazi murderous rampage did just that. Joseph and Mary did that as well when King Herod ordered the killing of newborns.

This state of being defiant (Iloabụchi) is extremely important because an individual's environment continually works as opposition-the law of opposition. Healthy and unhealthy competition can be considered 'opposition'. When someone goes for an interview and does not get the job, they could consider that the opposition won. In the case of a job interview, we can consider this healthy opposition because there is no penalty for not getting a job. By being in a state of defiance, the individual continues going for interviews until he lands a job. The defiance here is to unemployment or under-employment. It is a defiance of good over evil. Chiology is not about being a social deviant or defying society.

However, there are many cases of unhealthy and even fatal opposition. In the case of Martin Luther King, he was killed by the 'opposition'. However, his colleagues continued their 'defiance' and good won over evil.

The concept of 'Man is not the Chi' has another dimension. In some cases, people are in situations where they are beneficiaries. Some employees, girlfriends or boyfriends, housewives, etc could be in such situations. In this case, somebody else has become their Chi and determinants of their future. This is especially true of some women in abusive relationships who have no person to turn to, or no other place to go to. However, it is important that they understand that 'man is not the Chi'. They should endeavor to regain their Chi as soon as possible.

There is another principle in Igbo called 'onyebụchi' (which person is the Chi). It is another statement of defiance that suggests that another person is never another's Chi.

Summary

'Man is not the Chi' is a statement of defiance. This is an important way of being in Chiology. A Chiologist has a strong relationship with their Chi. They do not allow another individual to usurp their freedom and happiness indefinitely. It is important to confront or flee from oppressors.

Breathing techniques are very important in Chiology. The human body cannot remain alive without breathing. More importantly, the rate and depth of respiration is very important to anyone who seeks well being. We know that fast and shallow respiration is associated with anxiety and similar conditions, and other diseased states. In coherent breathing patterns, the plan is to achieve the opposite-calm breathing.

The Chi cannot be in its top form without a coherent breathing pattern. Coherent breathing is known to help eliminate stress and anxiety.

In Igbo, one of the ways to connect to the Chi and the Big Chi is through the breath. That's why the phrase 'kpọ kuo Chi-ukwu' is used when one intends to communicate to the Big Chi. Literally, 'Kpọ kuo Chi-ukwu' refers to 'call breath the Big Chi' or 'call the Big Chi through the breath'.

The lungs and healing.

The word for lungs 'ngụgụ' was derived from the verb 'gụgụ' which refers to 'healing' or 'consolation'. Simply put, we can use our lungs to console or heal ourselves. There is scientific evidence that when we slow our breath to about 3-6 cycles per minute, after 10 minutes, we begin to feel a sense of well-being. This is useful for stress, anxiety, depression, worry, post-traumatic stress disorder, phobias, physical and emotional pain, and respiratory problems. This breathing pattern is also very helpful for insomnia.

Spending time breathing at this relaxed rate is very helpful in connecting an individual to his/her Chi. A restless mind cannot readily connect to the Chi. This breathing pattern is known to lead to more relaxed and happy states.

Breath and Energy

The word for breath is 'ume' and is derived from the verb 'me' which is 'to do'. Obviously, we need to breathe if we want to do anything. Death is characterized by inability to breathe.

The word for energy is also 'ume'. Obviously energy is required to make thing happen. The Igbos use the same word for breath and energy because they are essentially the same concept. When we have shallow breath, we tend to have less energy. However, when we breathe slow and deep, our energy increases. We can safely state that breath is intimately related to our energy levels. The word for breath and energy are derived from the same verb 'me'(action) because both activities potentially yield action(s).

Further, the word for 'behavior' is 'u-me'. This is phonetically slightly different from the 'ume' of energy and breath. However the word for behavior 'u-me' contains the same verb 'me' (action).

It is easy to observe that our actions help define our behavior. This is because our breathing pattern affects our energy levels, which in turn has an impact on our actions. People whose behavioral patterns include fear and anxiety tend to have a different breathing pattern compared to those that are calm and confident.

Well grounded breath.

There's a phenomenon called 'umeana'. 'Umeana' can be considered as 'grounded breath'. Our breathing pattern affects our behavior. People who have a 'grounded breath' can be meticulous in their action(s). To achieve this state, one has to draw slow deep breaths to the extent that, metaphorically, the inhalation reaches the earth through the abdomen and legs. They can also practice slow deep breaths while lying on the earth (floor). Practitioners of this type of breathing achieve what has been called 'obi umeana' (the heart of the grounded breath). Such people have been described as peaceful, diligent, appropriate, highly productive, and generally well behaved.

Coherent breathing

'Ude' is a breathing pattern associated with an expiratory grunt. It is commonly observed in the elderly and children with severe malaria. It is characterized by a slow and deep inspiration, and an audible expiration. It is similar to the 'ujjayi' breath or coherent breathing seen in yoga and other eastern breath practices. 'Ude' could be a way to check the excess activity of the sympathetic (stress response) system, by up-regulating the opposing parasympathetic system. The sympathetic nervous system is responsible for secreting adrenalin and corticosteroids in preparation for 'flight or fight'. Chronic stimulation of the sympathetic nervous system, by stress or illness, is harmful to the body. 'Ude' induces wellness by increasing the activity of the opposing parasympathetic nervous system. Ude can be practiced as part of a healthy lifestyle in order to promote wellness.

For a CD that can guide an individual on Chiology breathing, please find the "breath energy" CD.

The relationship between breath, energy and behavior is well known in Yoga, Tai Chi, and other cultural healing methods around the world.

The Science of the Breath

It is well known that anger, stress, anxiety and other negative emotions can induce disease in organs of the body such as the gastro-intestinal tract. For example, pain and stress is known to increase gastric acid secretion that can lead to peptic ulcers. This is mediated through a complex bio-regulatory mechanism that involves hormones and the nervous system.

Impulses from diseased organs are carried via the vagus nerves to the interoceptive cortex where they are registered in the higher centers as subjective sensations of illness. The interoceptive cortex handles sensation from the internal organs, while the somatosensory cortex handles sensations that originate outside the body. The lung alveoli are rich in vagus nerve endings. When we slow and deepen our breaths to about 3-6 cycles per minute, more of the sensory nerves are activated. The impulses are carried via the vagus to the interoceptive cortex from where they are processed by the higher centers as subjective sensation of 'well being'. This helps explain how healing breath can make us feel much better.

Basically, healing breath helps counteract the effects of other negative emotions. When our Chi (personal guardian) contains more positive than negative emotions, we tend to have more success than failures.

In Chiology, awareness of the healing power of the breath is essential for longstanding happiness.

34

Step 5 Protecting the Chi

We know that Chi is related to the concept of God. God is the Big Chi. The Chi determines an individual's destiny, and the Chi is first. We also know the Chi is the lead. The leader is always well guarded. The US president is one of the most guarded persons in the world because of the importance of a leader. The same applies to the Chi. Every individual should protect their Chi with utmost zeal.

When an Igbo person is offended, they could say "maka Chi" which can be understood as "because of Chi". They could threaten to take a retaliatory action because of their Chi. They are not acting because of their body, but because of their Chi. We should be like that with our Chi.

In an abusive environment, our Chi is being harmed. Prolonged accumulation of negative energy in our Chi, by abuse, can lead to catastrophic results.

This means we should avoid and/or eliminate abusive people in our lives-for the sake of the Chi.

This calls for continued defiance of abusive people. One can keep vigilance on the condition of their Chi. Even the emotion 'shyness' should not be tolerated. The word for shyness is ife-ele. 'Ife' is 'something', while 'e-le' is 'inability to manifest'. Shyness in the Chi, is one of the factors that prevents us from manifesting our desires. For example, if you want a girlfriend you have to be talking to girls. Even if a girl blows you off in a public place, reconnect with your Chi and talk to the next girl. My advice is to talk to girls you consider very beautiful. The Chi is not heavily affected when one is blown off by a very beautiful woman.

Dance as a way to protect the Chi.

Dance is known as 'egwu'. Egwu was coined from the verb 'gwu'. 'Gwu' describes the digging motion that creates a mound and is also used in the word for hill (ugwu). The purpose of a mound is to protect a seedling or seed. In many ancient cultures, the hill is considered protective. The hill is protective against flood and fierce winds, and hills are easier to defend than open ground. The ancient people also considered dance a form of protection.

Dance and game are both known as 'egwu'. Dance is basically a game. The purpose of a game is to protect our spirit, so we can play more games. The Igbos understood that life is like a game with goals and obstructions. Although we may experience major painful events like losing a job, but life remains basically like a game.

Sometimes we get disillusioned, and give up our dreams and goals, because we have judged the barriers insurmountable.

We may feel like we are playing against a major football athlete and we have no chance of victory. Dance (egwu) is a game (egwu) that can rehabilitate and protect our spirit, so we can get back into the game of life. We naturally have a tendency to break into a dance when we score a goal in a sport (notice the hard work required to score a goal), because dance is naturally linked to achieving goals.

When we dance frequently, we would probably score more goals, in sports and in general life.

Dance is very good for the Chi (personal spiritual guardian).

Dance moves the Chi to more positive emotional states such as love and joy.

Games as a way to protect the Chi.

Life is a game and in life we ordinarily have goals. A general goal could be to live long. This goal, off-course, has several obstacles. It means we need to get a good job, have healthy relationships and eat healthy. Because life can be challenging, and we may not readily achieve our goals, and this may cost us some esteem. For instance, we may lose valuable people in our lives due to sickness and death. Naturally, these losses make us feel emotionally 'low'.

One way to protect our spirit, so we can keep playing the game of life, is to play games such as soccer or chess. These games expose us to the concept of win and loss in games, and all the emotions associated with it.

Games are good for the Chi.

Summary

Constant action is required to protect the Chi. This can be done with coherent breathing and movement procedures such as dance. Games help us protect the Chi so we can keep playing the game of good fortune. Sleep and rest is also very important in the game of life.

Step 6   No one is greater than their Chi

(Onyekachi)

It is important that people understand that no one is greater than their Chi. This is the basis of the statement 'onye ka Chi'. There are individuals who labor and labor but remain stagnant in life. It is their Chi. It is safe to assume that Saddam Hussein had murder, war and death in his Chi. No one can rise above their Chi. This is why the ancient people said "Chi-ji-ndụ"-the Chi holds life.

Even if an individual intervenes through breathing techniques, movement, or oiled perfumes, to raise their Chi, they still cannot rise above their Chi. They may record more successes and turn misfortune to joy, but they can never rise above their Chi.

The phrase "Chibụzọ"(Chi is first) is intended to remind us of this fact. An individual's Chi is always there even if the person is sleeping. When an individual awakens, their Chi is there. It is very important that individuals ensure that their Chi is in a good condition of love, happiness and exhilaration.

The Chi is of utmost important. One way of doing this is to have a favorable relationship with God- the Big Chi. Favorable here refers to a communicative relationship. In Christianity, it is written that we should put God first and other things will follow. This is also Chiology concept. To have a good Chi, one may have to cultivate a healthy relationship with the Big Chi, whether they are Christian, Muslim or Jewish, or any other religion.

Some Christian services start with singing and dancing-these activities are known to turn on more healthy emotions. Confession of sins is also powerful because it helps eliminate the guilt of sin. Guilt is a very powerful negative emotion. An individual cannot be happy if they are tortured by guilt.

Praying can be considered a way to accentuate desire so that one can act. Purposeful action can lead to happiness.

Especially important, is praying for others. Some people think they have the worst problems, but when they encounter a desperate person, they suddenly realize how lucky they are.

When an individual's Chi is in a state of love and happiness they are open, reasonable and energetic. This is a state that can lead to great accomplishment.

Summary

The Chi determines the position and fate of an individual in the society. Even if one intervenes through healing breath and other activities, one could record more successes, but cannot exceed their Chi.

No one is greater than their Chi. The Chi is the lead.

Step 7 Acknowledging Creation (Ekene)

Many people suffer from lack of satisfaction. They are constantly searching for a higher status. This robs them of the very important emotion known as satisfaction or contentment. Contentment is part of the spectrum of happiness. In African art, satisfaction is often depicted as a figure with a palm gently resting against the belly. A Chi without satisfaction is likely to be troubled. The word to greet or thank is known as 'Kene'. The Owerri people use a dialect that calls it 'kele'. It is derived from 'ke' (create or share) and 'ne' (to watch or acknowledge).

'Acknowledging creation' is an important way of acquiring emotional satisfaction. It is a way of expressing gratitude for being alive and well. This can be achieved by saying hello and some kind words to people you meet. By doing so you are acknowledging creation and obtaining a dose of satisfaction in return. Generally speaking, people naturally greet back when they are greeted. Powerful pulses of this emotion can be obtained when we do the greeting in a place of worship. In a place of worship, we are acknowledging a more powerful entity the 'big Chi'. In the olden days, it was done by bringing food items or animals to a Church or similar organization. In the western world, money is mostly used. There are clinical studies that show that people obtain more happiness by spending on others rather than on themselves. Satisfaction is a powerful emotion that stabilizes the emotions in the Chi.

If one wants to up the ante, they can do a bigger 'greeting' which can be called 'sacrifice'.

Summary

Gratitude is necessary to access emotional satisfaction. This can be obtained by greeting people, acknowledging the environment, or the Big Chi. In the modern world it can be done by giving money to a religious institution or charity of your choice.

Sacrifice in Ancient Igbo

Sacrifice is an important component of spirituality. Compared to Abraham whom God advised to sacrifice his son Isaac, we have it much easier. In modern times, we are often only required to sacrifice a small part of our income in terms of money.

People sacrifice huge sums of money to support the lavish lifestyles of some Pastors. Some are reported to own chauffeured Rolled Royce and private jets.

The only explanation is that sacrifice works for givers.

But why does it work?

The answer is in the ancient Igbo word for sacrifice 'ichụ-aja'.

This word illustrates the degree of sophistication of the extra-terrestrials that created Igbo (language). The word extra-terrestrial suggests that they are, literally, not from this earth.

'Ichụ' denotes to 'chase away' and 'aja' is from the verb 'ja' which is to 'communicate'. The sound 'a' is used to reverse the notion of communication making 'aja'-lack of communication.

Simply, ichụ-aja is chasing away 'lack of communication'. In other words, sacrifice (ichụ-aja) is 'enhancing communication'.

Sacrifice enhances our communication with the Big Chi that leads to His answers to everyday challenges. One of the properties of the Chi is to answer questions. It is captured in the phrase 'Chi-nasa' (Chi answers).

Sacrifice gives us an unprecedented ability to communicate with church leaders, church members and people in general.

The more you sacrifice (or give) the more you chase away negative communication.

Because an 'enhanced communication' is a state of being, which we can carry to our work places and businesses: it could result in success with money.

So don't expect the private jets to be grounded soon.

Sacrifice and walls

The 'aja' in sacrifice carries the same theme as the phonetically similar 'aja' (wall). A wall is a barrier to communication. With this new information, we may expand the definition of sacrifice to include the 'chasing away of spiritual walls' or the 'destruction of limitations'.

Sacrifice in the Judicial system

Crime is often committed by anti-social individuals. Part of the rehabilitation of these individuals is to mandate some form of community service. When these individuals sacrifice (or give), by fulfilling the 'punishment', it makes them more sociable.

On a scientific level, sacrifice (giving) is associated with increases in the pro-social hormones prolactin and oxytocin. These hormones are also released when we give and/or receive hugs.

Summary

Sacrifice through giving helps increase our ability to communicate. Enhanced communication with people, nature, and the Big Chi can help us have more happiness in our lives.

'Ike' is the word that represents 'strength' or 'power'. It is derived from the verb 'ke' that can be loosely translated to 'create'. To create is to put things together. A good creation provides some value to an individual, a family or the community. Power is required to put things together.

An individual who has negative emotions in their 'Chi' could be weak and may not have much valuable power. However, if they have love, happiness and similar positive emotions they could have more positive power. We know that God (Big Chi) is love, so an individual's 'Chi' in an optimal state should have plenty of love. Love creates a force of attraction between entities.

Some individuals have a lot of love in them. Some have a lot of love for their country and their people. Such individuals could strive to lead their country. They want to bring a better life for their people. When they succeed in an election, they could become very powerful.

Heads of corporate organizations could have plenty of power because they 'love' to have a diverse number of people use their products. Delivering services to millions of people could require thousands of supervisors and workers. Because the head of an organization manages supervisors and other workers, they could wield considerable power. This is how having plenty of love in ones Chi, can lead to power or strength.

Often, we notice that people abuse the power they have been given. Adolf Hitler abused the power he had, but we can't deny he had tremendous power. In my opinion, this is because hate and revenge in his Chi twisted his Chi and brought indescribable destruction to his people and himself.

However, a person with a 'good Chi' (Chi-ọma): could have tremendous power and can easily communicate with people. Such persons can get things done easily amongst 'right headed' people. This is why it is believed that Chinwike (Chi owns strength). This topic can be advanced to what is termed 'Chibuike'-Chi is strength.

In 'Chi is strength', we recognize that an individual's Chi is their strength. In the real world, a wide array of factors could sap an individual's strength. Everyday frustration and abusive people can turn a loving Chi into sadness, frustration and anger. However, coherent breathing techniques can be used to turn this around.

The bigger the love in a person's Chi, the more power they have. An individual can assess the size of their Chi by the number of people they can influence. The number of humans an individual influences is not the only measure of the size of the Chi. A farmer with 50 cattle has a bigger Chi than the one with 10. A game ranger responsible for the care of 50 trees, is more powerful than the one charged with one tree. These are general statements made on the assumption that all other conditions are equal.

We can easily relate that a reigning President of the United States would have a more powerful Chi than that of a small African country.

Summary

Our Chi is our strength. We have to ensure that it contains a lot of love in it. The proof of the strength is how many people our Chi can reach and influence, or how powerful we are in the community, and the physical universe including nature.

45

Sometimes we may have a job that does not require interaction with people. For example, a farmer can assess his Chi by the number of hectares he can cultivate and manage.

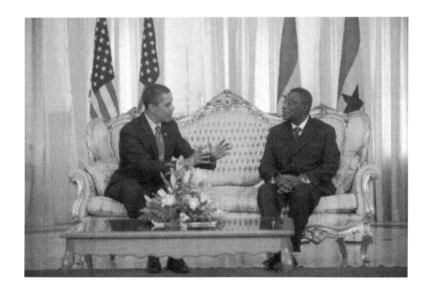

US President Barrack Obama and Ghanaian President John Mills.(Image by EPA/Shawn Thew). The phrase "onye ka mmadụ ka chi ya", suggests that 'a person can be greater than another individual and his/her Chi'.

Step 10   Chima (Chi knows).

Some people spend millions of dollars on clairvoyants, soothsayers and many other allied professionals. They want answers to their problems or misfortunes. Fortunately, the knowledge they seek is in their Chi, and the Chi of the people around them.

At the time of writing, a Malaysian Boeing 777 was reported to have crashed in the Indian Ocean killing all on board. The Boeing 777 has one of the best safety records, leaving many dumbfounded as to what could have happened to the plane. Until the flight data recorder is recovered, and the wreckage examined, we may never know what led to such a tragedy. Some suspect the pilots intentionally crashed the plane, others think it's a mechanical or electronic problem.

You may be shocked if I told you the cause of the air-crash is the Chi. The Chi is responsible for misfortune. This is because the Chi contains 'knowledge or expertise'. Regardless of the cause of the flight, theirs someone's Chi that contained incomplete or erroneous information. Even when an airplane is brought down by adverse weather condition, there's someone along the chain of safety that has inadequate knowledge of weather conditions.

Although flying is one of the safest modes of transportation, it is not risk free. Those who board planes have 'risk taking' in their Chi often without knowing it. Even in cases of mechanical failure, there were people in the airplane construction business that had incomplete knowledge in their Chi. Quite simply, whenever there's a disaster, it's the Chi. This summary is not intended to discourage people from flying but it is intended to extend the knowledge that flying is not risk free.

The individuals who came up with the idea of airplanes have risk taking in their Chi. Again, this monograph is not intended to discourage people from flying but people should recognize that any flight is risky, and anything can happen.

This is why Chiology recognizes 'Chi-ma'-Chi knows. Chi-ma is closely related to a similar subject termed 'Chineme'-the Chi is the doer.

When an individual has knowledge of something they can do something great. The 'ma' in Chi-ma is the word 'to know'. 'Ma' is also the word for 'good'. This is because knowledge is good, but also because to do something good, one requires knowledge. Surgeons have knowledge of the anatomy of the body, that's why they can do a good job inside the body.

Knowledge is one of the most important steps to happiness. An individual with poor knowledge of building cars will make a car that could crash and kill people. That would bring unhappiness to families and to the carmaker. The same thing applies to immigrants. Lack of knowledge of immigration laws brings misery to immigrants world-wide. Misery is obviously not good for the Chi.

One can acquire knowledge by simple observation, reading books, enrolling in a school or by other methods. Anyway, we look at it, knowledge is necessary for happiness. Knowledge brings us close to another quality of the Chi that can be called 'Chi-lota'. 'Chi-lota' means the 'Chi remembers' or the 'Chi can come up with information or ideas'. Whenever possible, we should let the Chi come up with information or ideas that can lead to solutions.

I know people who are good at their jobs but are unemployed. They were competent but they were either fired or laid off. It is not easy to say to them-"it's your Chi". There is something their Chi does not know. In some cases, their Chi has poor understanding of the economy, and they did not plan properly to changing fortunes in an industry. In some cases, their Chi has poor quality knowledge about humans. Bosses are known to fire rivals and keep their friends and psycho fans. It all boils down to relationships and knowledge of people. Racism and tribalism are real scourges that should be kept in the memory.

This is why some have said that Chi-ebuka (The Chi is very big).

Summary

The Chi contains knowledge. The Chi is responsible for disasters. A woman dies of childbirth because there's someone without knowledge of childbirth. Errors are caused by misinformation in the Chi. In the past, Polio was a problem globally. The collective Chi of scientists and doctors did not have a solution until the Salk and Sabin immunization was introduced. Today, in most parts of the world, Polio is history. So you can go to a remote village in India and I can show you someone who's Chi has the information that can prevent polio. All that is required is drops of the polio vaccination.

Step 11   Chi-di-ebele –The Chi is merciful

There are many problems in the world. Many die of starvation and disease. Millions live in misery and lack, and many take their lives because they cannot take it anymore.

Expectedly, there are many people who are highly spiritually and make it their business to help others. These people include helping others as part of the plan of their existence. There are some who have come to the realization that the only reason they want to live is to help.

Given the numerous and pervasive problem in the world, it is very reasonable that those who can help should do so. Ordinarily, there should be millions of people who dedicate themselves to helping others. These are the people of mercy.

Now in order to help or have mercy on others, one needs to have wealth. This is where the concept of 'Chinwuba' (the Chi owns wealth) comes in. Ideally, the reason the Chi acquires wealth is to give or help others. Each time we give, we can feel fulfilled because this is our purpose.

Summary

One of the properties of the Chi is mercy. The Chi is merciful to those in need, the poor, helpless, and the oppressed.

Step 12   Work as Revenge

Mbǫ -revenge

Mbǫlu-making revenge.

Revenge is a very important subject in every culture and spirituality. If we look at revenge in Christianity, we note that a certain action is prescribed. Moses had recommended an eye for an eye (tit for tat). This action must have been examined, and upheld, by many prophets that followed Moses like Jeremiah, Nehemiah, Elijah, and even John the Baptist. To the dismay of his fellow Hebrews, Jesus overturned the law and recommended 'turn the other cheek'. The action Jesus had recommended for revenge was the very opposite of 'tit for tat'. Jesus wanted us to show love to our enemies.

But how did the ancient Igbos consider revenge? What action did they prescribe as revenge? How should we revenge? The answer to that question lies in the Igbo word for revenge 'mbǫ'. Igbo as we know is a verb based language. The word mbǫ contains a verb or action word that denotes revenge.

Before we go into that verb or action word, I would like us to consider two closely related words. These words are closely related morphologically, semantically, and phonetically but are words for different subjects.

The first is 'mbǫ'; which is the word for nail(s).

The second is 'mbǫ'(phonologically different from the previous mbǫ) which is the word for hard or effective work.

So what do nails, effective work and revenge have in common?

How could these three entirely different subjects share a common motion or action?

To understand ancient Igbo: I would like to tell you a short story. You can call it a parable if you choose.

"In ancient times the Igbo were primarily an agricultural society; most people were farmers.

On one cool but sunny day, a prominent spiritual man was recalled to his house due to an emergency. As he approached his house, he noticed a small silent crowd. He was beckoned towards his house. As he entered, he heard moans and groans emanating from his bedroom. He walked closer, and as he opened the door he noticed a trusted friend on top of his wife.

Being spiritual and strong, he had a larger than normal hoe which he brought with him from the farm.

His grip hardened as rage diverted blood away from the centers of the brain that governed reasoning.

But from his Chi he heard the Igbo word for revenge; mbọ, mbọ, mbọ.

So he stepped back, turned around, and walked increasingly faster out of the house and towards the farm, and then he broke into a sprint. When he got into the farm, he dug, dug, dug, and dug. He enriched mounds, made new ones, and removed weeds. When he finished, the Sun was setting and when he looked at his farm it was very beautiful. It was as if he had made a new hairstyle on mother earth, and mother earth was smiling.

When he got back home, his house was empty. He was soon joined by a young lady who was very impressed by his action, and asked him why he did not kill the man, adding that "everyone would understand". The Nze (a shepherd priest) replied, "there is nothing to be impressed about". What I have done, today, has been repeatedly performed by men before me. He brought some palm wine out, and served the lady. "Chinyere (her name)" he said; "notice that I am not cleaning up blood, and I would not be facing the elders to determine if my actions are justified or not". "you see, our word for revenge mbọ is derived from 'bọ' which is the verb to dig". "We revenge by going back to work, to dig, and dig deeper. "That is the ultimate revenge", he said".

The verb bọ is used in the word for nail (mbọ) because the nail is used for digging (animals), or women use it to dig into the skin of their lovers. 'Bọ' is also the action word for hard work (mbo) because in an agricultural society, the only way to work effectively is to dig, dig, and dig (deeper)-digging out weeds that compete with crops for nutrients. Weeds are barriers to success.

In Chiology, a weed is any entity that can prevent an individual from attaining happiness. Weeds include family members, friends, acquaintances and colleagues- and need to be confronted or uprooted.

In Igbo, the prescribed action for revenge (mbọ) is to dig deeper into your work, digging out the barriers (weeds) to success; whether you are a farmer, doctor, lawyer, nurse or a shoe maker.

Chiology replaces a negative action that is associated with revenge with a positive action that can bring more positive emotions to our Chi. Revenge is a waste of time because it is a distraction from an individual's purpose. Happiness is a condition that is based on the ability to achieve long and short term goals. At the short term, this might seem counter-intuitive but on the long run, it is the right thing to do.

One of the first steps to happiness in Chiology is putting the Chi first. It is known as 'Chibuzo'. One needs to mentally connect to their Chi as they awake and ensure it is in a good state such as love and happiness. In such a state, thoughts of revenge should not have the upper hand. When an individual is fixated on revenge, it is a warning sign that their Chi is not in a good state. They should seek help by a registered professional.

There are two reasons we should not revenge. The first one is the common sense understanding that we also offend people by our actions when our Chi is not optimum. Secondly, people that act against us have very weak Chi and are going down anyway. It is not necessary to get involved in their woes.

The goals of a human being in a good mental condition should not include revenge against any group or person.

Revenge ravages the Chi because it is coupled with other negative emotions. In the above case, feelings of revenge would be accompanied by emotions of disbelief, anger, shock, distrust and a host of other negative emotions he must have experienced when he caught his wife cheating.

To be walking around with the emotions of revenge, is like taking your car for a service, but instead of ordering high grade motor oil, you ask for sand to be poured into the engine of your automobile.

Adolf Hitler is a perfect example of how revenge can wreak indescribable damage. The opposite of revenge is forgiveness. Forgiveness is no easy task, and requires mental homework. See forgiveness technology.

Once forgiveness is achieved, we can go back to our work and keep digging.

Chinazọ (the Chi saves) in revenge

In the modern world, there are laws that punish physical assault with several years in imprisonment. Some individuals are known to abuse this law by provoking vulnerable people to assault them. In another variant, some individuals misuse the controversial 'stand your ground' law, and use it as an excuse to murder innocent citizens.

One of the properties of the Chi is to ignore such provocateurs. In such cases, it should be recognized that the Chi can save someone from the misfortune of imprisonment. This phenomenon is also expressed in the concept of Chi-gbo (The Chi guards). This is why it is necessary to use breathing and movement techniques to encourage love and happiness in the Chi.

Summary

In Chiology, revenge is carried out by facing our purpose. Revenge is associated with other negative emotions such as hate, distrust, anger and disbelief. It is a big distraction that takes concentration and energy away from our true goals that could ultimately lead to happiness.

Step 13   Forgiveness

(Mgbahalu-leave things as is or live in the now)

Many people confess that forgiveness is very difficult. Sometimes a conflict has lingered for so long that forgiveness may seem impossible. Forgiveness between the Arabs and the Israelis may seem to be a far-fetched idea. Fortunately, forgiveness is something we must be able to do if we are to achieve health, love and happiness. While love and happiness are positive emotions, unforgiveness is a negative one. One of the features of love as recorded in 1 Corinthians 13 verse 5 is that it 'keeps no record of wrongs'. One of the reasons forgiveness is a challenge is because it requires active mental work. In Igbo, forgiveness is achieved by 'applying' the concept of 'leave it as is'. The key to forgiveness is to live in the 'now' or 'ugbua'. The reason we struggle to forgive is because we are not living in the now or present moment. For some reason, we keep going back to painful historic events. 'Ugbua' the word for 'now' was coined from the verb for pain (ugbu). The suffix 'a' is used to reverse the notion of pain making ugbua (now) as 'pain free'. To forgive, we may need to learn to live in the now. Coherent breathing can help an individual live more in the present moment rather than in the past.

Unforgiveness is one of the negative emotions that prevents an individual from remaining in the highest living state possible- the state of love. It is clear to many that forgiveness is more easily said than done, and it is understandably quite difficult to achieve. Other healthy ways of achieving forgiveness are therefore recommended.

One can engage in activities that turn on more positive emotions such as happiness and peace. Some of these activities are exercise, dance, singing, prayer, worship or studying the Bible or word of God.

Forgiveness is very good for the Chi. When we forgive, we get rid of negative emotions associated with unforgiveness. Forgiveness makes us feel better; much better than revenge. To forgive is to be the person you were pre-mental injury or emotional assault. To forgive is to recover emotionally and psychological to the point that you are who you were before the challenge. The experience acquired should prevent repeats of such infractions.

Anyone on this planet hoping to be well without forgiveness, might as well be wasting his/her time. Forgiveness is living.

In some tough cases of unforgiveness, Igbo forgiveness technology can be useful. Ichefu, ilofu, ilozọ and ichezọ are four methods of forgetting that can be useful in forgiveness.

Iche-fu (throwing away thoughts)

In this type of forgetting, a person is deliberately throwing away useless thoughts. This is a fully conscious individual, who is not suppressing or denying harmful thoughts. This is very useful in forgiveness. For example, a person practices throwing away negative thoughts, such as an experience with an abusive spouse.

Iche-zọ (to save or build a road in a thought)

The purpose of a road is to create a safe short-cut between two points. In Ichezọ, we deliberately jump from one thought to another by building a road in our thoughts. The intention is to by-pass painful thoughts or emotions. This type of forgetting is useful in forgiveness. For example, a friend of mine always remembers his ex-wife with some bitterness, so he learnt to build a road in his thoughts by remembering a period they were happy together. He would practice remembering her, then quickly go to a place they were happy together. He is quickly replacing a potentially depressing thought, with one with more pleasant sensations.

I know someone who was married for 20 years but is now facing a very painful divorce. He finds it very difficult to forgive his ex-wife. In his words, "the first 15 years of the marriage was good, while the last five was hellish". The strategy here is to think about the first 15 years and by pass the last five years.

If you were thinking: "oh this sounds like Jesus' love your enemy"-you are right! Hate is a negative emotion, that is very bad for the Chi. Building a way to more pleasant emotions in ones thought, is a practical way to love an 'enemy'.

Ilo-fu (throwing out a postulate)

In this higher form of forgetting, the spirit is responsible for the action. Here the spirit deliberately throws away 'negative thoughts' before making a postulate. This is very useful in forgiveness. In this case, a postulate does not include considerations from painful memories. For example, a woman says I like that tall guy, but tall guys always cheat. The postulate; 'tall guys always cheat' needs to be thrown away.

Ilo-zọ (building a road or saving a postulate)

In this type of forgetting, the spirit deliberately goes through a road in the memory lane in order to come up with a healthy postulate- bad painful memories are by-passed. This is obviously healthy for the mind and is good for forgiveness. For example, a woman was struggling to forgive her husband who crashed her car 6 months ago. Her husband borrowed her car 3 hours ago, and she says; "my husband is with my car and he is going to be here soon".

To have a good Chi, having a highly developed forgiveness technology is considered necessary.

Summary

Forgiveness is necessary for good health and a good Chi. Part of the difficulty in achieving forgiveness is a tendency to live in the past. When we learn to live in the present, we can readily leave the past behind and forgive.

Igbo technology of forgiveness involves exercises that involve throwing out and by-passing thoughts and postulates.

Step 14   Groups (O-tu)

Groups can provide some form of security. The feeling of security that can be obtained by joining a group is good for the Chi. A group also provides a forum for easy communication between members. Because the Chi has a mission, it seeks groups. A group can serve as a leveraging device: information can be easily disseminated through a group. Without adequate communication, it would be difficult for any one person to do much in the community.

In the Igbo language the word for a group is 'O-**tu**' and shares the same verb '**tu**' with the word for one (1) which is 'otu'. A group is a way to expand oneself into a much bigger entity.An active member of a group can easily leverage the collective power of the group. These very active members can be referred to as group leaders.

There are many groups that have benefitted humanity in incredible ways. Rotary International has a Polio eradication campaign that helped India eliminate the virus.

Summary

Joining a group provides emotional security and allows for more joy and happiness through success in ones goals and objectives.

Step 15 Healthy Lifestyle.

In Chiology, illness can be considered a misfortune. The Chi cannot be happy and loving when the body is ill. Since, Chiology is the study of love, the love of one's body should be an important directive.

There are many common sense ways of preventing illness such as eating well, getting adequate sunshine and physical exercise.

In animals, there is consistent evidence that restriction of calories in the diet prolongs survival. However, the evidence in humans is inconsistent and variable but there is general agreement that the body can be sustained on a low carbohydrate diet. Drs. Robert Atkins and John Salerno recommend that people should obtain most of their calories from proteins and healthy fat.

It is recommended that every individual get about 8 servings of fruits and vegetables daily. Adequate clean water is also necessary since the body is made up mostly of water. Consulting a registered nutritionist is wise.

Practically, some individuals are unable to obtain all the nutrients they need from the diet due to adverse lifestyles. Some of these individuals may have to resort to supplements.

According to US law, supplements are not to be used to diagnose or treat any disease. They can only be used for nutritional support. Some of the groups of supplements that may be necessary for healthy living are:

Multivitamins

Most vitamins are not made by the body and must be obtained from the diet. Some individuals, for variable reasons, may not obtain enough vitamins from the diet to sustain health. These individuals may have to resort to vitamin supplements manufactured and sold by reputable organizations.

Vitamin C is useful in tissue repair and has been shown to help boost the immune system.

Fish oil

Ideally, individuals should obtain fish oils from the diet, but this may be impractical for many people. Interest in fish oils arose after the observation of the low incidence of heart attacks in Eskimos who indulge in a fish rich diet.

Fish oils are Poly Unsaturated Fatty Acids (PUFA) and contain Omega-3 fatty acids. There are two distinct types of Omega-3 fatty acids; eicosapentanoic acid (EPA) and Docosahexanoic acid (DHA). DHA is abundant in the brain and eyes. Some clinical studies have shown that children who supplement their diet with DHA have improved test scores. However, it has not been conclusively proven that children should take DHA.

Fish oil has been shown to function as an anti-inflammatory agent and positively impact cholesterol and fat metabolism.

Body oils

The skin is the largest organ in the body and lotions and creams are recommended to keep it moist and healthy. It is, however, recommended that people should acquire beauty from the inside. A healthy life-style is necessary to achieve true beauty.

Another group of very important oils are the aromatic oils. An individual living in a foul smelling and unclean environment may have a hard time finding love and happiness. The sense of smell is carried by the first brain (cranial) nerve-the sense of smell is very important.

In his book "The interesting narrative of the life of Olaudah Equiano, it was mentioned that the greatest luxury of the Igbo was perfumes obtained from odoriferous trees. Part of the Chi enhancing strategy is good odor.

Aromatic oils can be dispensed with a diffuser or placed on hair or skin. Young living (www.youngliving.com) has a reputable brand of essential oils that are also edible.

Anti-oxidants

The process in which the body converts oxygen into energy produces oxygen radicals. The body has enzymes that can disable these radicals. However, there are occasions when the system can be overwhelmed and these radicals can damage the body's tissues.

There is some scientific agreement that these radicals contribute to the process of aging-the same way environmental exposure causes the rusting of nails. One of the main anti-aging doctrines is the heavy use of anti-oxidants. Ordinarily, anti-oxidants are abundant in fruits and vegetables such as broccoli and can be obtained from the diet. Anti-oxidants help in the mop up of excessive oxygen radicals.

In cases of inadequate dietary consumption, there are many supplements that contain berry extracts that have been shown to function as anti-oxidants. Vitamin C and red wine extracts are also powerful anti-oxidants.

Weight loss supplements

Obesity is a major problem around the world. People with a body mass index (BMI) greater than 25 but less than 30 are considered overweight. Those with a BMI greater than 30 are considered obese. Obesity is associated with hypertension and Diabetes Mellitus. These are conditions that can lead to serious health problems and early death.

Overweight individuals should consult a registered nutritionist. Calorie restriction and exercise are common recommendations, alongside a diet rich in fiber.

Again, supplements are not to be used to treat or diagnose any disease. However, some of the supplements recommended for weight loss include Garcinia cambogia, Irvingia gabonensis (African Mango), and Citrus aurantium (Advantra Z).

Digestive health.

The digestive system is important for a variety of reasons. Proper absorption of nutrients would be impaired in an individual with a sick digestive system.

The digestive system is also very important because it has a very rich network of nerves. It has been suggested that the digestive system has the second richest network behind the brain. More importantly, this network is very well connected to the brain. This is why certain emotional conditions are felt in the abdomen. Dr. Stephen Holt, MD in his book on Colon Hydrotherapy calls it the 'gut sense'.

A restive gut contributes to the emotional feeling of anxiety which is not helpful to the Chi. Gastro-intestinal irritants include certain foods and medicine should be avoided. Excessive alcohol is a well known stomach irritant. Non-steroidal anti-inflammatory drugs (NSAIDs) are a group of drugs that include agents such as aspirin and ibuprofen should also be avoided when possible. Patients who are deficient in the enzyme lactase, should avoid milk.

There are a number of agents that are known to support digestive health. This book is not intended to concentrate on supplements but probiotics are worth mentioning. Probiotics are gut friendly bacteria and yeast. They keep the overgrowth of harmful micro-organisms in check. Probiotics can be obtained from certain yogurt or raw kimchi. Kombucha, a special fermented tea, is also believed to supply gut friendly micro-organisms.

The Igbo obtained some of their probiotics from Ogiri which is fermented oil seeds.

Liver

The Igbo word for the liver is 'ume-ju' (full of energy/action). 'Ume' is a word that represents both 'energy' and 'action'. The liver is full of energy because it is the energy store house of the body. Energy is stored in the liver as glycogen. The liver is also the site of other body functions such as detoxification. Every highly active machine needs some type of maintenance. This is why the nutritional support of the liver should be considered. Milk thistle (Silymarin) should be considered as a detoxifier. However, I must reiterate that supplements are not to be used to treat or diagnose any disease.

Sleep

Sleep is a major part of a healthy lifestyle. Sleep deprivation is associated with anxiety, irritability, tiredness, and poor cognitive function. Lack of sleep has been shown to lead to premature aging, disability, obesity, impaired immune function, depression and death. In addition, sleep disorders have been shown to contribute to cardio-vascular diseases. Sleep problems cost the nation billions of dollars in lost time from work and tragic events, such as road traffic accidents. Sleep problems and death from automobile accidents is a classic example of how sleep problems can affect the Chi.

A healthy sleep lifestyle includes activities that help an individual wind down, such as light stretching exercises, reading a book, praying or meditation. Bringing work into the bedroom is not helpful. The bedroom is for sleep or sex.

When lifestyle changes fail to help with sleep, natural products can be considered. Again, these agents should not be used to diagnose or treat any medical condition.

Valerian root, chamomile flower, passion flower, lemon balm, Skullcap Whole, Ashwaghanda root, and catnip whole are some natural products used as sleep aids. See Clinical Sleep (www.naturalclinician.com)

Sex

Romance and love making is important in Chiology because it normally involves two individuals and their Chi. Sex is well known as an anti-aging tactic, and promotes good health. Sex is a broad and complex interaction that is not limited to penetration. Good sexual relationships encompass reinforcements of fore-play, penetration, and after sex activities. In Chiology, this can be supported with agreements between individuals. Couples can discuss their out-of-sync sexual activities and reach agreements on how to fix them.

Healthy sex is an important pathway to happiness. It provides an avenue for two people to have a healthy interaction that is gratifying and emotionally uplifting. Sex is an important way to impact positive emotions in an individuals Chi as well as in their partners Chi. It is a way to 'kill two birds with one stone'.

In the presence of sexual difficulties, natural methods are recommended as initial approaches. Lifestyle changes such as getting adequate sleep, frequent exercise, reduction or elimination of alcohol consumption are recommended to help ignite sexual arousal.

Natural and gentle supplements are recommended for individuals who may need them. Some of the agents used include arginine, muira puama, ginkgo biloba, tribulus terrestris, maca root, panax ginseng, and niacin.

Step 16   Cupping

(Chi reinforcement or Ichi Ochi)

The Chi determines an individual's position in the strata of life. A person who is considered successful in his/her community can be considered someone with a good Chi. 'Chi- ọma' (good Chi) is a concept that embodies the necessity of having a Chi full of love and happiness.

Physical and emotional pain, infectious diseases, and illness are some of the conditions that can be considered bad for the Chi. In the Bible, the lame were frequently targeted for miraculous work.

Musculoskeletal conditions can prevent an individual from working at full capacity and therefore has an impact on their Chi. The Chi cannot be loving and happy in the presence of pain and disability.

Cupping therapy is an ancient procedure that has been around for thousands of years. Cupping was described in the Ebers Papyrus, which is one of the oldest medical textbooks in the world, in 1550 B.C. Olaudah Equiano (c. 1745 – 31 March 1797) mentioned cupping as one of the Igbo practices in his book 'The Interesting narrative of the life of Olaudah Equiano'. In ancient times, the horns of animals were used. The horns had special valves that helped create suction. Currently, cupping is performed using plastic or glass devices. Suction is created by a mechanical hand-held pump or by an electric powered device.

There are two types of cupping: dry and wet. In dry cupping, there are no cuts on the skin. Wet cupping involves making incisions on the skin that leads to bleeding. Cupping is used in Chinese medicine to treat musculoskeletal conditions and respiratory diseases.

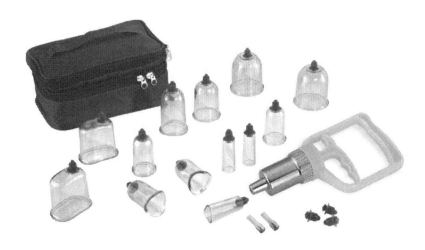

Cupping Kit. Image by Zkyl.

Summary

Cupping can be used to support the healing of respiratory, musculoskeletal and other conditions. Pain or physical debility is not helpful to the Chi. Disability can be considered a misfortune.

Step 17   Gentle Push (Owelle)

One of the worst things that can happen to the Chi is to be idle, have no job, have no goals, or have no plans to achieve a goal. Such a Chi can easily spiral downward into disaster and misfortune.

A Chi should always have goals. Dr. Nnamdi Azikiwe, the Owelle of Onitsha, who was the first president of Nigeria had a goal of making Nigeria great. His strategic plan was to make Nigeria a country others would envy. In order to achieve his goals, he had to enter politics so he can influence people. To influence people, his Chi had to reach agreements with their Chi.

In order to convert these agreements to actions and reality, a push is necessary. In order to achieve a gentle push, one must keep an eye on the heavens. The word for high or sky 'enu' is derived from the word 'nu' which is to 'push'. By looking at the heavens, we can be giving a gentle push of encouragement that can trickle down to others.

Sometimes we may be at loss on how to proceed. This is where the concept of Chi-nasa (Chi answers) becomes relevant. In such situations, all we have to do is to look up and ask the Chi. One of the properties of the Chi is the ability to answer. You can find out for yourself if this is real or not.

It is understandable that in Chiology, one of the necessary actions is to gently push ourselves and those around us. That is the easy way to achieve results. When things are easy we say it is 'wele wele'.

In Chiology, owelle is represented by flowing water. Upstream water causes movement of water downstream by gentle pushes.

Water trickling from the Fouta Djallon highlands in Guinea does not need to make a wild push to make water move towards the Niger Delta.

In Chiology, the aim is to push from above rather than from below. An objective initiated at the White House has a much better chance of success than one created at a slum.

Summary

Things are easier when we push from on top rather than from below. The strategy is to aim high and create a push from above.

Although wealth can bring an individual unbearable sorrow, it is generally agreed that having money is a good thing. Money can eliminate the frustration and pain associated with poverty. Pain and frustration can weaken an individual's Chi.

The Chi can be considered the 'end' of an individual, where he comes together, 'approximates', or comes to a 'head'. It can be considered a focal point, a summary, or complex in which the individual engages himself and the universe. If the individual engages more, they can have more. This ability to engage can be redefined as having the ability to reach others. Love and freedom are emotions that enable an individual play freely in the universe.

One important barrier to wealth is jealousy, especially when it is directed towards the rich. Jealousy is known as 'anya- ụfụ' and can be described as 'painful view'. In this condition, pain is distorting the view of the world. A jealous individual cannot see the real world and their vision is limited. Such as person, cannot easily reach out to others, especially the rich and happy.

To understand how the Chi brings wealth, one needs to picture an individual's Chi and its relationships with other peoples Chi.

73

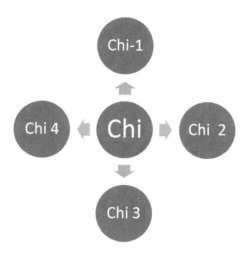

A persons Chi in relationship with other peoples Chi.

In summary, to have wealth, one must have a Chi that is healthy enough to provide a service or goods that can be exchanged. Then one must then interact with other individuals, whose Chi are big enough to exchange the service or goods for money. For this to happen, an individual must reach people. Advertisement can be considered a type of reaching out.

Poverty

The importance of reach is illustrated in the word for a poor person 'ogbenye'. Ogbenye was coined from 'ogbe'(section of community) & 'nye'(give). This is because a poor person is only given by a small part of a community. His/her reach is limited to a small part of a community. A person can be poor because he has a service or goods that are targeted to a small part of a community. On the other hand, wealth comes from having an extended reach- a Chi that reaches a wide number of other Chi's.

Wealth

Ordinarily, the only reason the exchange will occur is because their Chi wants the service or goods you are offering. The goods or services one is offering should be able to bring their Chi to a more favorable condition.

Even in cases of inheritance, the benefactor has a Chi that profits from the giving. In the case of military contracts, there are politicians and government officials whose Chi will be more at peace if contacts are awarded for defensive nuclear powered submarines.

In Chiology, wealth starts with having a product or service and then getting it to as many Chi as possible.

In order to reach many people, one needs to have a large capacity to make contacts and communicate with people. The word for wealth 'ụba' comes from the word 'ba' which means 'space' or 'entry'. The 'u' before 'ba' is a prefix used for community words. For details on Igbo prefixes on suffixes, please find 'Igbo voices: hidden wisdom from an ancient language' or 'Chi, and healing words from an ancient language'.

Things come from the Chi

'Ifesinachi' (things come from the Chi) is a very important concept related to the subject of wealth. Ifesinachi describes the concept that good or bad things come from an individual's Chi, and the Chi in his environment. Clean honest money is likely to come from an individual with good Chi.

This leads to a very important checklist regarding dealing with other individuals. It is important to note while dealing with people whether they have love and happiness or whether they are angry or spiteful. It is unlikely that healthy money can be obtained from an angry or spiteful person.

This also applies to making friends. People who are happy and loving are likely to help their friends become rich if they have substantial wealth.

At the time or writing, Walmart acknowledged that a good part of its income was derived from the US social security system. With this information, one might think that Walmart is getting rich off the Chi of the unemployed or partially employed. I suggest that Walmart is getting reach from the Chi of politicians and government officials who created the welfare system to help people in times of difficulties.

The concept of Uzọaga

Uzọaga is a principle that can be stated as 'no way' or 'there is no way there'. Wealth generation involves making investments or 'reaching out'. There are segments of the population that would not respond to ones wealth creating efforts. Stated another way, there are investments that will not bring the expected returns. These investments should be termed 'uzoaga'(there's no way there) and downsized or eliminated. Uzoaga is a way to save an individual or an organization wasted funds. Uzoaga is very important because the money saved can be regarded as income.

Summary.

The Chi owns everything (Chi-nwe), including wealth. Love and happiness is the key to true and healthy wealth.

Step 19   High Being (Ichi Echi-chi)

The last step is attaining a higher status. This phenomenon is termed 'Ichi echi-chi'. Notice the three Chis in that word. Now we know that the Chi is the personal guide of an individual. It is where the person ends, approximates, comes together, or comes to a 'head'.

We can translate Ichi echi-chi as a state of 'togetherness, togetherness and togetherness'. But because in its best form the Chi is love, we can also translate it as 'love, love and love'. Love is, off-course, a force that brings things together.

The proof of this is the fact that during a chieftaincy ceremony, there's a huge gathering. So how can someone be made to love, love and love?

The answer is also in the word 'Ichi echi-chi'. This is done by bringing the individuals Chi with the Chi in his environment.

The Chi in the community.

Assuming a high social status is a gradual and experiential process in which an individual begins to connect his Chi with his spouse and other people around him. This individual then bonds with family members, extended family, his community, his colleagues at work, etc. This can be considered a planned and deliberate unification of purpose. The phrase 'ndi ke mụ' is commonly understood as 'my people', but in Chiology it refers to 'people of my creation'. A high status person has a number of people who he agrees with, who are on his side, and who come to his defense in time of trouble. These people don't just show up, they are deliberately created through Chi agreements.

Unification of the Chi, starts with individuals the person agrees with, those he shares the same views with, or those he has things in common with. For example, a doctor can choose to draw near and unify with other doctors. These are individuals the person has some love for. The word for love 'Ifunanya' was coined from 'to see in the eye' or 'same view'. Love is tough when an individual has a spouse with a radically different view, or when an individual is a member of a community that wants to go west, when the individual wants to go east.

However, in a valued relationship it may be necessary to give up our own view in order to promote love.

Agreements

There's a specific method to marry an individual's Chi with the people around them. This is done through agreements or bonds. This is the basis of the famous saying; onye kwe Chi ya ekwe (when one agrees his/her Chi agrees). A couple can agree to move to Paris and their Chi will concur. A family could agree that there will be no infighting-and their Chi will concur. A group of people could decide to help the poor-and their Chi will concur. These agreements are the basis of the plea known as 'Chi-kwe'- let the Chi agree. These agreements or bonds can be verbal or written.

These agreements help an individual 'remain' in the right direction. These bonds and agreements can be useless in the absence of truth and justice. For example, one can agree with a merchant to buy a certain product for $20 each. If one can re-sell the item for $500, it may not be just to keep buying the item for $20 indefinitely. This is where truth and justice becomes important. Justice demands that the original agreement should be revised.

This is why an individual can be issued an 'ọfọ' which is a symbol of truth and justice. The ọfọ is a symbolic reminder that only truth and justice keep bonds or agreements. The word 'ọfọ' was coined from the word 'fọ' which is 'remain' or 'keep'. Commonly, the ọfọ is made from the branch of a special tree.

Agreements and bonds between humans are very important for a prosperous life. Formal agreements have been termed 'Igba ndụ' or 'life reinforcements'. Marriage between a man and a woman can be considered 'life reinforcement'.

Agreements with nature

Marrying the Chi with bonds and agreements is not limited to humans. A high status individual also marries his Chi with the plants and animals around him. He can also develop agreements that a certain tree will be kept and that a certain dog will remain.

Some individuals bond with birds such as the eagle and seek to conserve them. They could volunteer to protect the habitats of these great birds. Such an individual could choose to take an eagle (ugo) title. Ugo was coined from the verb 'go' which refers to 'esteem'. The eagle is a majestic bird that is often used as a symbol of power. One of the distinctions of a high status person is to create a bond, or become one, with a revered plant or animal.

Agreements with the heavens

Part of 'Ichi echi-echi' is to marry an individual's Chi to the heavens. This is why night fall and day break have Chi names which are Chi-ji and Chi-fo respectively. These are periods an individual could recharge their Chi with breathing and movement techniques. Aligning the Chi with these celestial activities is very important. An alignment with the sun (anwụ) is also very important. Anwụ was coined from the verb 'nwụ' which is 'to die'. The prefix 'a' is used to create the negative, making 'anwụ' that which 'does not die'. Life is not possible without the sun.

'Anyanwụ'(eye for the sun) is another distinction that keeps an individual aware of the position of the sun in the heavens. It helps orient an individual to his position on earth. Alignment to the moon, and stars is also necessary. The strategy is to plan to start projects at a new moon (new moon ceremony), and to observe the movement of starry bodies.

Summary

Attaining a higher status (Ichi echichi) is characterized by 'marrying' a person's Chi to his family Chi, the community, the environment and the heavens. The 'marriage' is done through agreements or bonds and held in place by truth and justice. The 'ọfọ' is a symbolic reminder that only truth and justice keeps bonds and agreements.

The marriage of the Chi's is dynamic and an individual learns how to operate these relationships. Breathing and movement techniques are important operational tools. Knowledge of how to operate the Chi has been termed 'Ife chi'. 'Ife chi' has been interpreted as 'worshipping the Chi' but it can be more accurately described as 'flying the Chi'.

Now you have some knowledge and some tools-you can make your Chi 'fly' through love and happiness.

Conclusion

Chiology is a way to happiness based on ancient and current Igbo culture. It begins with the recognition that everyone has a Chi, and the need to put the Chi first.

One of the most important ways of being in Chiology is 'defiance' based on Iloabuchi (a postulate that man is not the Chi). Iloabụchi and mmadụabụchi (man is not the Chi) are tools that can be used against oppressors.

Breathing and movement techniques can be used to protect the Chi, and promote love and happiness.

To gain a higher status, one has to learn to marry the Chi to the Chi in his family, community, environment, and heavens. Agreements and bonds are used to bring different Chi together, and these arrangements are maintained with truth and justice.

Skillful management of Chi relationships could give an individual the necessary power to achieve their goals, and also empower them with the ability to handle future goals. Happiness can be considered a condition in which an individual has learnt the knowhow to handle life challenges.

The Chiology way to happiness introduces many of these happiness tools.

The End

Chiology will return as Advanced Chiology.

BIBLIOGRAPHY

1. Aguwa, Jude C. U. (1995). *The Agwu deity in Igbo religion*. Fourth Dimension Publishing Co., Ltd. p. 29. ISBN 978-156-399-0.
2. Basden, George Thomas (1921). *Among the Ibos of Nigeria.* Nonsuch Publishing
3. Botha, R. and C. Knight (eds) 2009. *The Cradle of Language.* Oxford: Oxford University Press.
4. Chikodi Anunobi. Nri Warriors of Peace. Zenith Press; 1 edition (February 28, 2006)
5. Chinua Achebe. Things Fall Apart. Anchor Books -- Doubleday, NYC (January 1, 1994)
6. Chinua Achebe. No Longer at Ease. Heinemann, 1960.
7. Chinua Achebe. Arrow of God. Heinemann, 1964.
8. Chinua Achebe. There was a country: a personal history of Biafra. © 2013 Penguin.
9. Christopher Ejizu. Ofo; Igbo ritual and symbol. Fourth Dimension Publishing Co. (March 11, 2002).
10. Davidson, R and Begley S. The emotional life of your brain: How its unique patterns affect the way you think , feel and live-and how you can change them. © 2012 Plume.
11. Dr. Creflo Dollar. Experiencing God's Love. A guide for new believers. Creflo Dollar Ministries ISBN 1-59089-806-0.
12. Eckhart Tolle. The Power of Now: A Guide to Spiritual Enlightenment. New world library, 2004
13. Eckhart Tolle. A New Earth. Awakening to your Life's purpose. Penguin, 2008.
14. Frantzis, Bruce Kumar . *The Chi Revolution: Harnessing the Healing Power of Your Life Force*. Blue Snake Books. ISBN 1-58394-193-2.
15. Frey Bruno S Happy People Live Longer, , Science 4 February 2011: 542-543.

16. Gallup. State of the American Workplace Report 2013.

17. Holt, Stephen. Combat Syndrom X, Y, Z. Wellness publishing (2002).

18. Holt, Stephen. A certification program for dietary supplement councilors. Holt Institute of Medicine press © 2008. www.hiom.org

19. Holt, Stephen. The definitive guide to colon hydrotherapy: Principles and Practice of Colonic Irrigation. © 2013 Holt Institute of Medicine.

20. Holt, Stephen. Sleep naturally. © 2003 Wellness publishing.

21. Holt, Stephen. Sex the natural way.(c) 2011 Holt Institute of Medicine.

22. http://en.wikipedia.org/wiki/Shalom

23. Ilogu, Edmund (1974). *Christianity and Ibo culture*. Brill. ISBN 90-04-04021-8

24. Isichei, Elizabeth Allo (1997). *A History of African Societies to 1870*. Cambridge University Press. p. 247. ISBN 0-521-45599-5.

25. Iwu, Maurice. *Handbook of African medicinal plants*. CRC Press; 1 edition (February 18, 1993).

26. Kanno T, et al. Peptic ulcers after the Great East Japan earthquake and tsunami: possible existence of psychosocial stress ulcers in humans J Gastroenterol. 2013 Apr;48(4):483-90.

27. M. O. Ené "The fundamentals of Odinani"

28. http://www.kwenu.com/odinani/odinani.htm

29. Nwosu CD, Ojimelukwe PC. Improvement of the traditional method of ogiri production and identification of the micro-organisms associated with the fermentation process . Plant Foods Hum Nutr. 1993 May;43(3):267-72.

30. Nwosu, Uzoma. Igbo voices; hidden wisdom from an ancient language. © 2013

31. Nwosu, Uzoma. Chi, and healing words from an ancient language. © 2013

32. Ogomaka, P.M.C, (in press), 'Number Systems including some Indigenous Number Systems'. Teaching Modules for Secondary School Teachers of General Mathematics, Abuja: NMC

33. Ogomaka, P.M.C. & Akukwe, A.C., 1998, 'School and Work place Mathematics in Imo State: Some implications', Nigerian Journal of Curriculum and Instruction, Vol. 7, No 1:13-18

34. Ohuche, R.O, Ezeilo, J.O.C; Eke, B. I, et al., 1986, Everyday Mathematics for the Junior Secondary School, Book 1, Enugu: Fourth Dimension Publishers.

35. Olaudah Equiano, *The Interesting Narrative of the Life of Olaudah Equiano, or Gustavus Vassa, the African.* Simon & Brown publishers.

36. Onwuejeogwu, M. Angulu (1981). *An Igbo civilization: Nri kingdom & hegemony.* Ethnographica. ISBN 978-123-105-X.

37. Opata, Damian U. Ekwensu In the Igbo Imagination : a Heroic Deity Or Christian Devil, Nsukka, Nigeria : Great AP Express, 2005.

38. Pamela J. W. Gore (1996-01-22). "Phases of the Moon". Georgia Perimeter College. http://facstaff.gpc.edu/~pgore/astronomy/astr101/moonphas.htm

39. Patrick Mathias Chukwuaku Ogomaka. Traditional Igbo Numbering System: A Reconstruction. Africa Development, Vol. XXX, No.3, 2005, pp. 35–47 © Council for the Development of Social Science Research in Africa, 2005 (ISSN 0850-3907)

40. Richard P. Brown M.D. and Patricia L. Gerbarg. The Healing Power of the breath. 2012 Shambhala publications.

41. Salerno, John P. The Salerno Solution. © 2013 Take Charge books.

42. Sylvester Okwunodu Ogbechie,: *Ben Enwonwu: the making of an African modernist*. University Rochester Press, 2008.
43. The Holy Bible.
44. Uchendu, Victor C. *The Igbo of Southeast Nigeria*. Van Nostrand Reinhold Company, 1965.
45. Udeani, Chibueze C. (2007). *Inculturation as dialogue: Igbo culture and the message of Christ*. Rodopi. p. 28—29. ISBN 90-420-2229-9.
46. Uzukwu, E. Elochukwu (1997). *Worship as body language: introduction to Christian worship : an African orientation*. Liturgical Press. ISBN 0-8146-6151-3.

Books and publications by the Author.

1. Kenneth A. Egol, M.D., Jaspal R. Singh, M.D., and Uzoma Nwosu, M.D. Functional Outcome in Patients Treated for Chronic Posttraumatic Osteomyelitis. Bulletin of the NYU Hospital for Joint Diseases 2009;67(4):313-7.
2. Jaspal Ricky Singh, M.D., Uzoma Nwosu, M.D., and Kenneth A. Egol, M.D. Long-Term Functional Outcome and Donor-Site Morbidity Associated with Autogenous Iliac Crest Bone Grafts Utilizing a Modified Anterior Approach . Bulletin of the NYU Hospital for Joint Diseases 2009;67(4):347-51.
3. Uzoma Nwosu, MD. Igbo voices; hidden wisdom from an ancient language. ©2013
4. Uzoma Nwosu, MD. Chi, and healing words from an ancient language © 2013
5. Stephen Holt MD, Uzoma Nwosu, MD, Clifford Carroll. The Topical Pain Relief Revolution: Principles and Practice of Compounding Pharmacy. © 2013 Holt Institute of Medicine.

About the Author.

Dr. Uzoma Nwosu is a graduate of College of Medicine, University of Nigeria, Enugu Campus. He worked as a Principal Medical Officer with the department of Health, Johannesburg, South Africa before joining the Pharmaceutical Industry to perform research. Dr. Nwosu also worked as a Research Fellow at the NYU Hospital for Joint Diseases. He is a co-author of peer-reviewed medical papers.

He is keenly interested in African culture, and its impact on human health and development. The decision to write this book was made after reading the book "Nri Warriors of Peace" by Chikodi Anunobi. Subsequently, an analysis of the Igbo word for lungs, 'ngugu' showed it was coined from the verb 'gugu' which means to console. This discovery led to Dr. Richard Brown and his wife Dr. Patricia Garberg, who teach the use of breath in Healing.

This helped validate the many thoughts behind Igbo words and accelerated the development of this book.

Index